Unshackling the Past

A Guide to Healing Childhood Trauma

Janice Sheilah, Cheryl Guan, Lidia Leong, and Sam Choo.

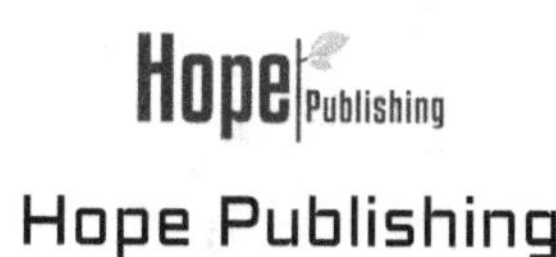
Hope Publishing

Hope Publishing

Contents

Chapter 1

Childhood trauma is a topic that is near and dear to my heart, which is why I felt compelled to create this book. I believe that it is an invisible mental disease that can limit our growth and potential by weighing us down with memories of the past. Many of us struggle with doubts and limitations that we impose upon ourselves, and these can often be traced back to our childhood experiences.

For instance, I personally have a fear of failure that often prevents me from trying new things. This fear stems from the fact that in the past, I was scolded and punished whenever I made mistakes. However, I have come to realize that in order to learn and grow, we must be willing to make mistakes and take risks.

Furthermore, I have noticed that I often seek approval from others because I never received compliments or positive reinforcement during my childhood. This realization has helped me to better understand myself and my behaviors.

In addition to my own experiences, I have also witnessed the impact of childhood trauma on my daughter. She has struggled to let go of past hurts and memories, and I have prayed that this book will help others who are in similar situations and cannot seem to move on with their lives.

While I do not claim to be an expert on this topic, I have invited three of my friends to contribute their stories and perspectives to this book. Each of them has written a chapter, and their diverse views and experiences are sure to enrich and inspire readers. From recognizing the signs and symptoms of hidden trauma to exploring the roots of our childhood experiences, this book covers a wide range of topics aimed at helping readers overcome their past and thrive in the present and future.

Here's a teaser of what we will be sharing:

Janice Sheilah:

Discover one woman's journey of overcoming a tumultuous childhood marked by toxic family situations, and how she turned her experiences into lessons of growth and renewal. In this powerful and inspiring article, Janice Sheilah shares her story and provides hope for others seeking to heal from childhood trauma. Join her as she navigates the challenges of her past, and learn how you too can transform your own experiences into a brighter, more resilient future.

Cheryl Guan:

Discover the power of self-help tools to overcome overwhelming emotions, and learn how to reclaim your self-worth and self-esteem with the guidance of Cheryl Guan, a Licensed Therapist and Shamanic Healer. In this insightful article, Cheryl shares her journey towards self-discovery and the practical techniques she used to build a healthier, happier life. Gain control over your emotions and find purpose and inner strength as you take the first steps towards transforming your life with these effective self-help methods.

Lidia Leong:

Discover the key to healing your inner child and unlocking your full potential. Learn about the common types of childhood wounds, the traits of co-dependency, and the practical steps you can take to heal your inner child. Lidia shares her personal journey and offers guidance on how to release trapped emotions, set healthy boundaries, and embrace self-love. It's time to embark on your own healing journey and unveil the unique gifts that lie within you.

Sam Choo:

Get ready to embark on a journey of self-discovery and healing with this comprehensive guide on overcoming childhood trauma. In this writeup, you'll explore the invisible scars that trauma can leave, learn how to identify hidden signs and symptoms, and delve into the roots of your own trauma. You'll also discover how trauma affects relationships and explore strategies for healing and building resilience. With a focus on forgiveness, vulnerability, and community, this guide will equip you with the tools you need to thrive beyond trauma and help loved ones on their own healing journeys. Join us as we explore the lifelong journey of growth and healing.

Chapter 2

Growing up, I never experienced any significant personal trauma; however, my family wasn't perfect, and I had to navigate some toxic situations as a child.

One of the most prominent toxic situations in my family was the constant fighting and arguing between my parents. It seemed like every other day there was a new disagreement or argument that would escalate into a full-blown fight. As a child, it was incredibly scary and confusing to witness the two people who were supposed to protect and love me the most acting in such a volatile and unhealthy way. I remember feeling like I was constantly walking on eggshells, never sure when the next argument was going to happen or what it would be about

In addition to the constant fighting, there was also a lack of communication and emotional intimacy in my family. My parents rarely talked to each other or to me about their feelings or any issues they were facing. Instead, they would bottle everything up until it erupted into an argument. This lack of communication made it difficult for me to feel connected to my parents or to understand what was happening in their lives.

Another toxic situation I experienced as a child was the lack of boundaries and respect for personal space. My mom would often invade my privacy by going through my things without my permission. She would also constantly criticize and nitpick at me, making me feel like I could never do anything right. This lack of boundaries made it difficult for me to feel safe and respected in my own home.

Despite all of these toxic situations, I tried my best to focus on the good things in my life and find ways to cope with the negative aspects of my family. I found solace in my hobbies and activities, such as playing the piano and drawing. Additionally, I made sure to surround myself with positive and supportive people, such as my older sister, who helped me feel valued and loved

Looking back on my childhood, I realize that while my family wasn't perfect, I was able to learn valuable lessons from the toxic situations I experienced. I learned how to manage and cope with difficult emotions, such as anger and sadness, and how to communicate more effectively with others. Additionally, I learned the importance of boundaries and respect for personal space, and how to set and enforce those boundaries in my own relationships.

While I can't change the past, I can use my experiences to create a healthier and more positive future for myself, my daughter, and those around me. I strive to be more mindful of the way I communicate and interact with others, creating a safe and supportive environment for myself and my loved ones. Additionally, I work to be more understanding and compassionate towards others who may be going through difficult or toxic situations, knowing firsthand how challenging it can be to navigate them.

Overall, my childhood wasn't perfect, but it has shaped me into the person I am today. While I wouldn't wish toxic situations on anyone, I believe that we can all learn and grow from them if we approach them with a positive and open mindset.

Childhood trauma can have a profound and lasting effect on one's life, leading to a range of negative outcomes such as difficulty forming and maintaining relationships, low self-esteem, and mental health issues, including depression and anxiety.

The good news is that it is possible to overcome childhood trauma and lead a healthy, fulfilling life. An important step is to seek support from a therapist or counselor to help you process and work through the trauma. It may be beneficial to join a support group or seek out other resources and information about how to cope with trauma.

In addition, taking care of your physical and emotional wellbeing can be crucial in healing from trauma. You may want to practice self-care activities such as exercise, meditation, and engaging in hobbies or activities that bring you joy. It is also important to find healthy ways to deal with stress and emotions, such as through deep breathing, journaling, or talking to a trusted friend or loved one

About Janice Sheilah

Janice Sheilah is a travel enthusiast, writer, and artist. She loves exploring new places, capturing her experiences through words and drawings, and sharing them with others. You can follow her on Twitter @janicesheilah to see her latest travel adventures and creative projects.

Chapter 3

How to Let Go of Overwhelming Emotions and Find Inner Strengths

After nine years of marriage, Deborah and her husband had been longing for a child, but had not been able to conceive. In desperation, Deborah prayed to Mary, Mother of Jesus, to grant her a child. Miraculously, her prayer was answered, and Deborah was soon pregnant with me. She always said I was a miracle baby, as I was a gift from God.

Many people assumed that I had been a spoilt child due to being an only child, and that my parents had supposedly doted on me. Although I wished this was the case, my childhood had been a harrowing experience instead. For a long time, I had sought to reassure myself that I had been a blessing to the family.

When I was born, my mother Deborah had to go to work, leaving me in the care of my maternal grandmother, Esther. Everyone in the family was intimidated by her, as she was a strict dictator. My aunt Lucy and her two sons, Caleb (3 years old) and Joshua (5 years old)

also lived with Esther after the passing of my uncle, Lucy's husband. Most of the time, Lucy was away working, so she was rarely home.

Esther was an avid gambler and liked to invite her friends over for mah-jong sessions at her house. She would also sometimes visit her neighbor's place to enjoy a game. Despite her hobby, she never neglected Caleb, Joshua and I, and was given a monthly allowance from Deborah and three of her other children.

Esther's emotions were often unstable, fluctuating in a very short span of time on most days. Whenever she lost money gambling, she would become furious. Similarly, she would become frustrated if we were unable to meet her expectations. Even small things could get her boiling, and she would direct her anger at us through caning, scolding, and shouting.

Growing up, Esther was psychologically and emotionally abusive towards me and my cousins. From the age of four, I was subjected to endless statements such as, "You're a jinx to the family, and your parents don't want you!" Hearing these hurtful words from Esther for ten years had a strong impact on me, and I began to internalize them, believing them to be true.

Deborah was aware of Esther's cruel behavior, yet she stayed quiet out of fear. She minimized Esther's violent actions and reassured me of Esther's love. Although Esther and Deborah both claimed they loved me, their actions contrasted their words.

Every day, I lived with a sense of dread, never knowing when Esther might become unhinged over the most minor issues, such as using the wrong colored clothes peg for laundry. The struggle was mine to bear, as my father, Samuel, saw it as Deborah's responsibility to manage Esther's unacceptable and violent behaviour and refused to get involved.

On my way home from school one day, I felt overwhelmed with despair, believing that my presence in my family was nothing more than a source of anguish. My pain became so unbearable that I even had thoughts of suicide, more specifically, jumping off the block of flats.

Suddenly, an angel appeared before me, a being of pure white. It was tall, with broad wings that shimmered in the sunlight, and a halo of light around its head. The sight of the angel and its quick disappearance brought me feelings of peace and comfort, as though it had been sent to reassure me in my time of need.

At the age of 12, when I was considering ending my life, I saw the angel again. This time, it lingered for a moment, filling me with a sense of warmth and peace. It was then that I realized that I had a purpose in this world, that there was a reason for me to be here. The angel's appearance gave me hope and strength, and helped me to overcome my despair.

I was determined to take control of my life and make the best of it. To cope with Esther's unstable moods, I adopted various strategies such as blocking out her negative words and immersing myself in sports. Running became a form of therapy to help me release my turbulent feelings. I also diverted my focus to my studies and successfully attained my bachelor's degree from Monash University.

At the age of 12, I moved back to stay with my parents permanently. My paternal grandmother, Julia, also resided with us. Despite my parents still having to work, they believed I was old enough to take care of myself while under the supervision of Julia. On weekends, I slept over at Deborah's place. They trusted me to be responsible and took steps to ensure my safety.

Even though the atmosphere in my parents' house was peaceful, the lack of engagement between Julia and me was suffocating. I would play by myself and watch television. My parents were never outwardly verbal or physically expressive, and yet their love was palpable through the delicious meals they provided. Every Saturday, my dad would take me out to get dim sum before dropping me off at Esther's place. Despite this, I still felt a disconnect in terms of the emotional bond that I had with my parents.

Impact of Childhood on Adulthood

Since the age of 21, my childhood traumas have had a large impact on my adulthood. I developed low self-esteem and felt that I wasn't worth anything. I believed that anyone who got close to me would be cursed. As such, I put an emotional wall up between myself and those around me. Despite this, I was still praised by my former bosses and colleagues for being responsible, diligent, and hardworking. I was often able to work for long hours without feeling exhausted.

When I saw that my friends and ex-colleagues could express their emotions easily, I became aware of my own inability to do the same. This worried me, as I was a social work associate helping clients and families cope with difficult situations. In order to empathize with them and provide meaningful assistance, I knew that I had to understand my own feelings. Thus, I decided to seek counseling.

I was experiencing symptoms of Complex Post-Traumatic Stress Disorder (PTSD). This disorder is often the result of prolonged exposure to traumatic events, especially during youth. Symptoms of Complex PTSD can include anxiety, depression, social isolation, difficulty forming relationships, and difficulty regulating emotions.

The counsellor pointed out to me that I had disconnected from my emotions at the age of nine as a way to protect myself from my difficult environment at the time. While this method of coping was helpful at the time, it had a big effect on me over the years.

After my first counseling session, I decided to actively observe my emotions each day. However, I initially found it hard to do so and I felt discouraged when I could not respond emotionally to people who wanted to help me.

At first, it was difficult for me to access my emotions. However, with time, I gradually became more in tune with them. After a few sessions with a counselor, I was able to put names to my feelings, such as happiness, anger, sadness, and disappointment.

As an adult, the difficulties my parents and Esther faced in providing care for me and my cousins became clearer. My parents confided that they had not felt an emotional connection to their own parents, while Esther was in an unfavorable marriage. Her husband failed to contribute to caregiving or provide financially, meaning that Esther had to work long hours to ensure that Deborah and her three younger siblings had food and shelter.

Being the eldest, Deborah had to take on the responsibility of helping Esther take care of her siblings, having gone through a tough childhood herself. Meanwhile, John, my father, was mainly taken care of by the maid of his parents.

Julia led a quiet life. She was an introverted individual and did not need to be around the children much. She typically kept to herself instead of interacting and playing with them. Her husband, Albert, was the sole breadwinner of the family. He spent many hours at work and had no time for his children. John modeled himself after Albert for being a diligent and reliable husband and father who provided for the family.

Even though my parents never vocalized how much they loved me, they showed their love through their actions. My mother would often bake and cook the food that I enjoy eating, while my dad would buy the food that I like. I also tried to develop my relationship with them by engaging in activities that were of interest to them. Over time, this allowed me to forgive both my parents and Esther, enabling me to continue living my life.

Growing up, I endured experiences that resulted in me developing strong fear and anxiety. When I was working as a counselor and helping those exhibiting explosive and violent behavior, these anxieties worsened. Even though I had the knowledge and skills to successfully assist such people, the constant tension in my body became increasingly intense.

I went for my second round of counseling, but unfortunately, I did not find it to be useful. Verbal conversations were not enough to help me reduce my fear and anxiety. I was taught the Eye Movement Desensitization and Reprocessing (EMDR) method to cope with my anxiety, however, the results were only temporary.

Despite attending a breakthrough course to help me break free from self-limiting beliefs, painful challenges, and move towards the desired outcome, I found myself experiencing irrelevant fear. I did the guided activities, experienced outbursts of emotion, but my fear remained.

Following a friend's recommendation, I decided to take part in a course on family constellations. This therapeutic process helps to unravel disruptive patterns in families, such as unhappiness, illness, and addiction. I felt that joining an experiential course was the best way to acquire the knowledge and skills required, as well as having the opportunity to work on my own issues. Therefore, I chose to take the course, and I am confident that it will be beneficial for me.

During my constellation process, interestingly, I became aware of a generational fear instead of childhood pain. Upon further investigation, I found out from my mother that during World War II, she had been close to death when a bomb dropped near her. Thankfully, Deborah, my maternal grandmother, was alert and able to rescue her in time. Though the course was helpful, and individual coaching was available after the course, I found the sessions to be too expensive. I did not engage the coach for any coaching sessions.

Desperately seeking help for my anxiety, I explored many different avenues, including counseling and breakthrough courses, but to no avail. As a result, I began to search for alternative methods of treatment and soon discovered Shamanism. Through this Google search, I hoped to find a solution to my struggles.

While visiting Singapore, I discovered that shamanic practitioner Teya E Star brings the powerful and transformative modality of shamanism to help people release emotional traumas, obstacles, and burdens, as well as outdated beliefs that may be preventing them from becoming the highest version of themselves.

The shamanic healer was able to uncover deep-rooted fear stemming from childhood experiences without me having to provide a narrative and helped me to reach my desired outcome.

I was five years old when I witnessed my aunt attempting to throw my cousin, Caleb, out of the window. The memory of this traumatic experience came flooding back when I was told that my fear of being harmed started after that incident. I remember becoming less talkative afterwards, indicating a deep fear and worry. Energetically, I also felt that I had not fully forgiven Esther and my mother for what had happened.

I knew in my logical mind that forgiveness was the right thing to do, but deep within, I was still unable to let go of the anger I held towards them. My unresolved trauma had a profound effect on my emotional development.

At 34, when I sought help from Teya, I felt emotionally immature due to a unique phenomenon known as soul loss. In shamanic terms, this happens when a person experiences physical or emotional trauma, whereby a part of their soul lives in the timeline of the traumatic event. In counseling, it is referred to as "soul fragmentation".

During my healing sessions, I experienced a profound emotional release of anger, hatred and sadness. My body trembled and I felt nauseated, as if a heavy rock was being removed from my heart. I could finally breathe more deeply and felt a newfound sense of ease. I am feeling lighter, both energetically and emotionally, after my pain has been released.

I have been amazed by the shamanic healing method and motivated to use the most effective methods to help my clients break free from years of agony and achieve their goals. This led me to pursue a Shamanic Practitioner training course, and I have since been using this modality to help many clients reach a core transformation in the shortest amount of time possible. Remarkably, I have seen such success that often only two shamanic healing sessions are required.

Effects of repressed emotions

Many people try to bury their pain and move on as if nothing has happened, using methods such as working long hours, watching TV, exercising, smoking, and drinking alcohol. Unfortunately, this leads to repressed emotions moving into the unconscious, where they can be triggered by similar situations or someone who says or does something upsetting. This can have adverse effects on our health. When seeking help, it's essential to recognize that these unprocessed emotions need to be addressed and dealt with properly.

As adults, we are in control of how we want to live our lives, even if our pasts cannot be changed. Self-blame and blaming others can only lead to misery, so it is important to discover and focus on our purpose in life. Doing this will help us break free of any self-limiting beliefs or practices that may be holding us back and provide an inner strength and joy to propel us forward. With purpose and goals firmly in mind, we are more motivated to break free of those things that hold us back.

It was a challenge to rewire my beliefs about myself, but I was able to do it through consistent practice with self-help tools. I'm happy to share the tools that helped me work through self-doubt and value my worth.

Self-help Tools

To increase self-worth and self-esteem, here are 8 healthy ways to cope with and release overwhelming emotions:

#1: Writing: Take a piece of paper and write whatever comes to your mind. There's no need to second-guess or question your thoughts and emotions. You don't have to write in complete sentences, as only you will read what you wrote. Once you're done, tear the paper into pieces and discard it.

#2: Earthing: Spend 15 minutes walking barefoot on grass. This can help reduce stress levels, as grass absorbs lower frequency energy from the body, leading to a calming effect and increased relaxation.

#3: Grounding: Use a stainless steel spoon to massage the bottom of your feet for one minute each. Rub the curved side of the spoon against your skin to stimulate and ground your body. You can test the spoon's material with a magnet - if the magnet sticks, it's made of stainless steel.

#4: Nature: Take a walk or jog in nature, consciously breathing in fresh air and letting go of anything that is overwhelming you. Focus on this practice for 10 minutes to experience a relaxing effect.

#5: **Shower**: Fill your bathtub or basin with water and add a few drops of lavender essential oil and a cup of Himalayan sea salt into it. Soak yourself for 10 minutes in the bathtub if available and for a few minutes in a basin. Rinse off the salt water afterwards.

#6: **Light Bath**: Find a peaceful place to sit comfortably and close your eyes. Imagine a beam of bright, pure white light from the heavens or from a higher power streaming down to the crown of your head. Visualize this divine light filling your body, from your head to the tips of your toes. Allow this light to sweep away any discomfort or blocks from the deepest parts of your being, and see them leaving your body and entering the Earth beneath you.

#7: **Screaming and Crying**: Screaming and crying help to energetically release pent up emotions. You can scream into the pillow, shout to the sea or cry in your private space.

#8: **Dance**: No dance expertise is necessary to experience the therapeutic effects of expressive movement. All you need is a song of your liking and let your body lead you in whichever way it desires. Create a private space for yourself and let the music take you away to explore the freedom of movement as a form of self-expression.

#9: **Body Scan**: Find a place where you can be free from distractions and allow yourself to relax. Close your eyes and focus on any undesired emotions that you may be feeling. Ask yourself, "Which part of my body am I feeling this emotion in…?" Place one hand on that area of your body and take your time to experience and express the emotion. If you find yourself wanting to scream or cry, use a pillow to muffle the sound. Let go of the emotions and take your time.

#10: **Sleep**: Having difficulty sleeping can be frustrating, however, taking some time to create a calming bedtime routine can help you drift off to sleep. Set the mood by playing some calming music, then begin to count backwards from 100 slowly before you doze off.

If you want to reclaim your self-worth and self-esteem, here are 10 useful tips to help you do that:

1. Take some time to recognize your talents and qualities. Ask your family and friends to help you identify your strengths.

2. Don't forget to reward yourself for every success you achieve.

3. Help someone in need to make yourself feel good.

4. Before you sleep, take a moment to appreciate yourself for who you are.

5. Look at yourself in the mirror and tell yourself that you are important and loved.

6. Check your self-talk; if you find self-criticizing thoughts, stop them immediately and replace them with more positive thoughts.

7. Begin to say "no" when you do not really want to.

8. Forgive yourself if you make mistakes and be kind and gentle

to yourself.

9. Write down something at the end of the day that you are proud of.

10. Take time to pamper yourself and make sure to treat yourself with love and respect.

About Cheryl Guan

Cheryl Guan is a certified counsellor, social worker and shamanic healer. She specializes in providing counseling and therapy services to individuals and families who are struggling with emotional and psychological distress. With her expertise in understanding the unique needs of her clients, Cheryl strives to empower them to build strong and healthy relationships. She also promotes self-acceptance and self-worth, guiding her clients towards a happier and more fulfilling life. You can learn more about Cheryl's services at .

Chapter 4

What is the Inner Child?

The inner child is the part of our psyche that developed during childhood and continues to live within us. It represents our younger self and carries memories from our early experiences, including how we learned to process information from our environment.

While some childhood memories may be positive, others may be painful and difficult to deal with. It is often these painful memories that linger in our subconscious and lead to self-limiting beliefs.

Parents and caregivers play a crucial role in a child's emotional well-being and development. Unfortunately, many parents were not equipped with the necessary tools to support their children's emotional growth. This can result in a child's emotional maturity not progressing with their age. As a result, the inner child can become stuck with painful memories from ages 5 to 11, and some may even carry trauma from before birth without realizing it.

What affects the Inner Child Psyche

Conditioning and Perception

As children, we are taught certain values and beliefs by our parents or caregivers. However, these values and beliefs are not always based on truth, but rather on societal norms, education, and past generations. Our parents were also influenced by their own upbringing and conditioning.

The values and beliefs we adopt from our parents or caregivers can shape our personality, habits, patterns, attitudes, and mindset. However, we have the power to change our beliefs and rewire our minds. The way we perceive and receive love from our parents may also differ from their intentions.

For example, a child may feel unhappy with tough love from a strict mother, while the mother believes it is necessary for the child to learn discipline and obedience.

In another scenario, a busy father may have little time to spend with his family, creating a sense of an "absent father." The mother may feel neglected without her husband's love and concern, and this may impact her ability to fully nurture and love the children, leaving them feeling neglected as well.

<u>Shadows and Generational Trauma</u>

Parents and the generations before them may carry unhealed traumas and wounds that they unknowingly project onto their children. As children see their parents as role models, they learn from their behaviors and absorb their energies, often taking their parents' narratives as truth.

Shadows are the parts of ourselves that we deny, repress, or suppress. When someone triggers our shadows, we may either repress or react to them.

Generational trauma refers to wounds passed down from earlier generations who experienced tragedies such as wars, poverty, hunger, the Great Depression, economic crises, addictions, substance abuse, and family violence.

There are several ways that inner child wounds can manifest, but they generally fall into seven main categories:

1. Abandonment

2. Neglect

3. Perfectionism / Low Self-worth

4. Guilt

5. Distrust

6. Abuse

7. Co-dependency

1. Abandonment Issues

Children may experience abandonment when their parents leave them or entrust them to other caregivers. This can lead to feelings of being unwanted, undeserving of love, unworthy, unloved, and unlovable. Children may grow up feeling isolated and lonely, with a fear of being left alone, left out, or excluded. This can lead to co-dependent behavior and a pattern of attracting emotionally un-available relationships. In adulthood, these feelings can create a lack of commitment in romantic relationships.

2. Neglect Issues

Children may experience neglect when their parents do not give them enough attention or love in the way they desire. This can lead to feelings of inadequacy, unworthiness, repressed emotions, fear of vulnerability, and a tendency to get angry easily and struggle to let things go. Children may grow up adopting these behaviors, which can attract people who make them feel invisible or unheard.

3. Perfectionism/Low Self-Worth Issues

Children may develop perfectionism or low self-worth when one of their parents is very demanding, harsh, or strict on their development and growth. Children may grow up in an environment where they are pressured to participate in many enrichment classes and excel in all areas. As a result, they may feel that they are not good enough or worthy, always needing to achieve something new or better.

Children may grow up to be competitive high achievers, seeking accolades and awards to feel seen as good enough. While this may appear as self-confidence, their subconscious may still be seeking to improve themselves because they feel something is lacking.

4. Guilt Issues

Children may develop guilt when caregivers manipulate them with threats, emotional blackmail, or guilt trips. This can result in children feeling unable to ask for assistance or set boundaries, making it difficult to say no. As a result, they may become people-pleasers, allowing others to take advantage of them.

If the child is the eldest, parents may put heavy responsibilities on them from a young age and not provide them with enough love and nurturing. This can lead to the child carrying this belief throughout their lives, prioritizing the needs of others and neglecting their own emotional needs.

5. Distrustful Issues

Children raised in an environment of criticism, distrust, and insecurity may become victims of emotional abuse, which can have a detrimental effect on their emotional growth and well-being. As a result, they may be constantly afraid of being hurt, judged, or rejected, and have difficulty trusting others, themselves, and their own judgment.

This can lead to seeking external validation from others and attracting people who also have difficulty trusting. With low self-esteem and lack of confidence, they may find it hard to rely on their own gut instincts and inner voice.

6. Abuse Issues

Children raised in a physically abusive family may feel unsafe and develop unhealthy coping mechanisms. This may include exerting dominance over others or struggling to set and maintain boundaries for themselves.

7. Co-dependency Issues

Children raised by narcissistic parents or parents who are overly or under-protective may be susceptible to developing various inner child wounds, such as guilt, perfectionism, low self-worth, and distrust. These issues can lead to co-dependency.

Traits of Co-dependency

- Care-giving and over-worrying for others

- Controlling or trying to fix/correct others

- Always giving unsolicited advice

- Perfectionism

- Unable to ask for help or unable to accept help

- Self-critical

- Guilt; feeling responsible for everybody and everything

- People-pleasing

- Ignoring your own needs or wants at the expense of others

- Always seeking external validation and approval

- Overworking and extending yourself to the point of burnout

- Difficulty with open communication, vulnerability, and intimacy in relationships

- Emotionally reactive or sensitive to criticisms

- Anxiety or depression

- Feeling that you are being taken advantage of.

How to heal the inner child wounds

Inner child wounds are stored memories in the emotional body, which consists of the heart center, abdominal area, and pelvic area. Here are eight ways to heal inner child wounds.

1. Journaling. You can connect with your inner child by journaling. Write down any event that you still have memories of that provokes strong emotions such as anger, sadness, resentment, jealousy, or a sense of unfairness.

Try using your non-dominant hand to write down the event; it may trigger emotions or tears. Sit with these emotions and allow any release to flow.

Be present in the moment and be aware of how you feel. Be kind to yourself during the process of releasing these emotions.

Acknowledge that the past is already gone, and there is no need to hold onto these memories. Set the intention that you now allow these memories and emotions to be released for good.

2. **Inner Child Mediation.** You can connect with your inner child through meditation or age regression to help you recall memories, heal, and release painful emotions. As a therapist, I conduct Inner Child Healing Meditations to help my clients connect with their inner child.

To reparent your inner child, hug them and be present for them. Tell them that you love them and give them your attention and love as the type of parent that you would have wanted.

3. **Play.** If you feel like you grew up too fast and missed out on the joys of childhood, find ways to reconnect with your inner child. Engage in activities you missed in your childhood or hobbies that bring you joy. Allow your inner child to be creative and have fun.

4. Art Therapy. Use art as a form of therapy for your inner child to express themselves freely, without restrictions or minimal guidance. This exercises the right brain hemisphere of creativity and inspiration, allowing for free expression. Most education systems are too rigid and restrictive, confining brain function to be left-brain logic-focused. Art therapy gives you the space for free flow of expression.

5. Creative Projects. The healed inner child can be very creative and inspirational. Engage in creative projects that utilize its natural creative juices to produce art in various forms or mediums, such as writing, designing, painting, singing, dancing, playing musical instruments, crafting, or creating innovative inventions.

6. Emotional Freedom Tapping (EFT). EFT is a tapping technique that methodically activates nine meridian points to reconnect with traumas held in the body and release them. You can find more information on accredited EFT Tapping Training with EFT International (https://eftinternational.org/).

7. Setting Personal Boundaries. Acknowledge that you deserve to be loved and respected. Be assertive and stand your ground. Clearly communicate your needs and wants to others. Don't worry about offending others - your feelings and opinions matter!

8. Practicing Self-Love and Self-Care. Love and accept yourself for who you are, and be authentically you. Be kind and compassionate to yourself, and don't judge yourself too harshly. Take care of your physical and mental well-being; get enough rest, exercise, and eat healthily. Reconnect with nature by going for walks. Adopt a new activity such as meditation, yoga, jogging, tai chi, kickboxing, or something that interests you. Don't let the criticism of others affect you; use your wisdom to decide if it's useful information or something to discard.

Processing the Inner Child

Wounds

It's important to understand and process our inner child wounds. As children, we weren't taught how to manage our emotions and thoughts correctly, and our parents were often unable to understand what we were thinking and feeling. This left us to manage our emotions and thoughts alone. However, as adults, we are better equipped to understand what we went through in a more mature and informed way. It's essential to illustrate examples of the different types of traumas to help us better understand and process our emotions and thought processes. External circumstances beyond our control or our parents' control can also influence how we are affected.

1. Abandonment Wound

Some parents may abandon their children due to poverty or their inability to afford the costs of raising them. This may be their last resort, either abandoning them to an orphanage or one of the parents leaving the family.

2. Neglect Wound

One of the parents being the sole breadwinner may have resulted in insufficient time and attention given to nurturing the children or providing them with sufficient emotional support.

3: Perfectionist Wound

Some parents may have high or harsh expectations of their children to excel in all areas of life, including academics, sports, or artistic pursuits. Children may be subjected to attending various classes to learn multiple activities in order to excel in every area.

This places tremendous pressure on young children to learn quickly in a short period of time, without considering individual learning speeds and abilities. It cultivates a perfectionist wound that one must constantly learn to meet their parents' expectations and earn their validation, as well as collecting awards and accolades to prove their worth to the world. Without these achievements, they may feel worthless and judge others without them as less worthy.

The child may grow up to be a perfectionist, scrutinizing small, petty things they deem imperfect or flawed. In some cases, this may develop into Obsessive-Compulsive Disorder (OCD), although not always. As adults, they may become very demanding in their jobs and relationships.

4. Guilt Wound

Some parents use guilt as a tool to get their children to comply with their demands. They may make their children feel guilty for not doing what they want or not meeting their expectations, which can lead to a sense of obligation and an inability to say no or set boundaries. This can result in a lack of assertiveness and a tendency to prioritize the needs of others over their own, which can lead to feelings of resentment and self-neglect. As they grow into adulthood, they may struggle to set boundaries or assert themselves, and may continue to seek external validation and approval.

5. Distrust Wound

The development of trust begins in the first 15 months of life. Through physical contact, bonding with their parents, and the energy they can sense from them, an infant begins to form the basis for trust. If a parent is distrustful, skeptical, or critical, the infant's process of learning trust can be disturbed, and they may grow up to be distrustful of relationships and themselves. This can lead to the avoidance of long-lasting or committed relationships and the rejection of relationships or potential partners out of fear of being hurt or rejected.

6. Abuse Wound

When children witness family violence happening within the household, either to a parent or to themselves, it can have a significant impact on their mental, emotional, and physical well-being, which can be very traumatic.

It can also happen in the case of parents with substance abuse, addictions to alcohol, gambling, and other vices, causing the children to feel that the family environment is unstable and unhappy to live in. This can also create a deep distrust of relationships, feeling unsafe and insecure without the love and support of healthy living conditions.

They may be unable to form healthy relationships and may be prone to attracting people who abuse them, or they may become abusers themselves as a form of trauma response in fighting mode.

They may become hypersensitive to physical touch, entering a fight, flight, or freeze mode.

7. Co-dependency Wound

In the scenario of a narcissistic parent, the child felt controlled and restricted, leaving them feeling like a victim. This could lead to them growing up with low self-esteem, a lack of feeling worthy of love, and a reliance on being rescued by somebody else. Alternatively, they may grow up to become a martyr, rescuing and fixing others in order to make themselves feel needed and validated.

Traumas can only be released through releasing the trapped emotions from the body. Talk therapy-style coaching is not totally effective in releasing emotional traumas because it does not penetrate to the emotional level of the subtle body, which is essential for healing.

The healing of the inner child can be a long and on-going process, depending on the depth and number of layers of wounds present.

As each layer of trauma and wound is released and healed, you can experience yourself feeling lighter and more able to feel joy and delight. You will also be more able to express yourself freely, uninhibited, and authentically while sharing your gifts with courage to the world.

In every shadow lies a gift. The shadow is simply a gift that is obscured from the light. When we start to accept our shadows, we acknowledge that perfection is not the goal. We are here to be unique, weird, funny, loud, quiet, to take up space and much more. It doesn't matter what others think of us. What matters is how we view ourselves and how we live according to that view. We can make a difference in the world simply by being ourselves, regardless of how small or large an impact it may have.

The meaning of life is to find your gift. The purpose of life is to give it away

About Lidia Leong

Lidia Leong is a spiritual life coach, energy healing therapist, and a student of metaphysics. She is devoted to healing her own inner child and helping others to heal theirs, so that they can access their power and express their unique gifts to the world while leading joyful, blissful, and abundant lives.

www.empathyhealings.com

https://youtube.com/EmpathyHealings

Chapter 5

It was a beautiful, sunny day, and Sarah had just left the office, feeling excited about the upcoming weekend. As she walked towards her car, she couldn't help but feel a tight knot in her stomach. She tried to shrug it off, but the uneasy feeling persisted. Even though there was no apparent reason for her anxiety, it was always there, lurking in the background like a shadow.

Sarah's story is one that many people can relate to. In fact, it's quite possible that you, too, have felt a similar unease without being able to pinpoint its origin.

That's where "Unshackling the Past: A Guide to Healing Childhood Trauma" comes in. This book is designed to help you uncover the hidden wounds of your past, shed light on their impact, and guide you on a path toward healing and self-discovery.

Understanding Childhood Trauma

Childhood trauma is often referred to as the "invisible wound" because its effects are not always immediately apparent. It can manifest in subtle ways, influencing your thoughts, emotions, and behaviors without you even realizing it. But what exactly is childhood trauma? Simply put, it is any distressing or harmful experience that occurs during childhood, leading to lasting emotional pain and psychological distress.

Imagine a young boy named Jack. Jack was only seven years old when his parents got divorced. As a child, he couldn't fully grasp the complexities of his parents' separation, and he felt overwhelmed by the intense emotions that came with it. Jack's parents, consumed by their own pain, were unable to provide the emotional support he needed. As Jack grew older, he developed a deep-seated fear of abandonment, which affected his relationships and self-esteem throughout his life.

The Purpose of This Book

"Unshackling the Past" is a guide to help you recognize, understand, and heal from the invisible scars of childhood trauma. Throughout this book, you'll find personal stories, practical advice, and gentle encouragement to guide you on your journey toward healing.

Every person's experience with childhood trauma is unique, and so is their path to healing. This book is not meant to provide a one-size-fits-all solution, but rather to offer you the tools and insights you need to embark on your own journey of self-discovery and growth.

Perhaps you're like Sarah, experiencing anxiety without knowing the root cause. Or maybe you're like Jack, struggling to understand the impact of a painful event from your past. Regardless of your experience, this book is for you. It is for anyone who is ready to uncover the invisible scars of their past, heal their wounds, and embrace a brighter, more fulfilling future.

So, take a deep breath, and let's begin this journey together. We'll start by exploring the signs and symptoms that can indicate the presence of hidden childhood trauma. As you read through the following chapters, keep an open mind and be gentle with yourself. Remember, healing is a process, and it's never too late to begin.

I'd like to share a story with you about a woman named Emily. Emily was struggling with depression and anxiety. She had tried various treatments and therapies, but nothing seemed to help. As we began to explore her past, it became clear that Emily had experienced significant childhood trauma. Together, we worked through her painful memories and emotions, and over time, Emily began to heal. The dark cloud of depression that had hung over her for so long gradually began to lift, and she started to continue rediscover her inner strength and resilience.

Emily's journey wasn't easy, and there were many moments when she doubted herself and felt overwhelmed. But she persisted, and with each step she took, she became more connected to her authentic self. As she learned to embrace her vulnerability and face her past with courage and compassion, Emily's relationships improved, and she began to experience more joy and fulfillment in her life.

Emily's story is just one example of the power of healing childhood trauma. It is my hope that, through this book, you too can find the strength to face your past and begin your own journey toward healing and self-discovery.

Healing is not a linear process, and it can often feel like taking two steps forward and one step back. It's essential to remember that progress comes in many forms, and even small steps can lead to significant growth and change. As you move through this book, I encourage you to be patient with yourself and celebrate each small victory along the way.

In the coming chapters, we'll delve deeper into the various aspects of childhood trauma, helping you recognize the signs and symptoms, understand the roots of your trauma, and explore how it may be affecting your relationships. We'll also discuss practical strategies for healing, such as developing self-compassion, seeking support, and establishing healthy boundaries.

But before we dive into the specifics, let's take a moment to acknowledge the courage it takes to embark on this journey. Facing your past and healing from childhood trauma can be a daunting and vulnerable experience, but it is also an opportunity for tremendous growth and transformation.

So, as you read through "Unshackling the Past," remember that you are not alone. There are countless others who have walked this path before you and found healing, and there is a community of support available to help you along the way. And most importantly, remember that you are deserving of love, happiness, and a life free from the invisible scars of your past.

Let's continue this journey together, gently uncovering the hidden wounds of your childhood, learning from the wisdom of your experiences, and ultimately, embracing the unshackled future that awaits you.

As you progress through this book, remember to be kind to yourself, and trust that with each step you take, you are moving closer to healing and a more fulfilling life.

Chapter 6

As we delve into the world of hidden childhood trauma, it's essential to recognize that its effects can manifest in various ways. Sometimes, the signs and symptoms may be subtle, making it difficult to connect them to past experiences. In this chapter, we'll explore some common indicators that may suggest the presence of unresolved childhood trauma, helping you identify any hidden wounds that may be affecting your life.

Emotional Indicators

One of the most common ways that childhood trauma can manifest is through emotional responses. These might include feelings of anxiety, depression, fear, or anger. Let's look at the story of Jake, who struggled with feelings of anger throughout his life.

Growing up, Jake was constantly yelled at by his father. As a child, he internalized his father's anger, which later manifested as bouts of unexplained rage. Jake's unresolved trauma led to strained relationships and difficulties at work.

If you find yourself experiencing intense emotions that seem disproportionate to your current circumstances, it may be a sign that unresolved childhood trauma is affecting you.

Behavioral Patterns

Childhood trauma can also influence our behaviors and the way we interact with the world. Here are some common behavioral patterns that may be linked to unresolved trauma:

Self-sabotage: People who have experienced trauma may unconsciously sabotage their own success or happiness. For example, Amy, who grew up with a neglectful mother, may struggle to maintain healthy relationships as an adult because she fears being abandoned again.

Perfectionism: Those who have experienced trauma may develop perfectionistic tendencies as a way to regain control over their lives. Consider the story of Sam, who was constantly criticized by his father. As an adult, Sam became a perfectionist, fearing that any mistake would result in rejection or criticism.

Avoidance: Unresolved trauma can lead people to avoid situations that trigger memories or emotions related to their past experiences. For instance, if Lisa was bullied at school, she might avoid social situations as an adult, fearing judgment or ridicule.

Cognitive and Physical Clues

In addition to emotional and behavioral signs, unresolved childhood trauma can manifest in cognitive and physical symptoms. Some examples include:

Memory lapses: Traumatic experiences can be repressed or forgotten, leading to gaps in memory or difficulty recalling certain events from childhood.

Intrusive thoughts: Individuals with unresolved trauma may experience intrusive thoughts or flashbacks related to their past experiences, even if they are not consciously aware of their trauma.

Physical symptoms: Unresolved trauma can manifest as physical symptoms, such as headaches, stomachaches, or unexplained aches and pains. These symptoms might be your body's way of signaling unresolved emotional pain.

As we explore these signs and symptoms, it's important to remember that they do not automatically indicate the presence of childhood trauma. However, if you recognize several of these indicators in your own life, it may be worth considering whether unresolved trauma could be playing a role.

It's also important to note that everyone's experience with trauma is unique, and the signs and symptoms can manifest differently for each person. As you read through this chapter and the rest of the book, remember to be gentle with yourself and trust your intuition. If something resonates with you, it may be worth exploring further on your journey to healing and self-discovery.

Chapter 7

Understanding the origins of your childhood trauma is an important step in the healing process. By exploring the various factors that may have contributed to your past experiences, you can gain valuable insights into the patterns and beliefs that have shaped your life.

In this chapter, we'll discuss some common sources of childhood trauma, including family dynamics, adverse childhood experiences (ACEs), and the role of school and peers.

Family Dynamics and Parenting Styles

Our family environment plays a crucial role in shaping our early experiences and emotional development. Different parenting styles and family dynamics can contribute to childhood trauma. Some common examples include:

Authoritarian parenting: Parents who are overly controlling or demanding can create an environment in which children feel constantly criticized or afraid of making mistakes. This can lead to feelings of shame, low self-esteem, and anxiety.

Emotional neglect: Parents who are emotionally unavailable or unresponsive to their children's needs can create a sense of worthlessness and a deep-seated belief that love is conditional.

Dysfunctional family dynamics: Families that are affected by addiction, mental illness, or domestic violence can create a chaotic and unpredictable environment, leading to feelings of insecurity and instability in children.

Adverse Childhood Experiences (ACEs)

Adverse childhood experiences (ACEs) are specific traumatic events that can have long-lasting effects on a person's emotional and physical well-being. Some common ACEs include:

Physical, emotional, or sexual abuse: Abuse can have a profound impact on a child's sense of safety and self-worth, often leading to feelings of shame, guilt, and self-blame.

Parental separation or divorce: The loss of a stable family structure can create feelings of abandonment and insecurity, particularly if the separation is accompanied by ongoing conflict or tension.

Witnessing violence or experiencing a traumatic event: Exposure to violence or trauma, such as a natural disaster, car accident, or the death of a loved one, can leave a lasting impact on a child's emotional well-being.

The Role of School and Peers

While family dynamics and adverse experiences are significant contributors to childhood trauma, it's important to recognize the influence of school and peers as well. Some common experiences that can contribute to trauma include:

Bullying: Being the target of bullying can lead to feelings of isolation, fear, and low self-esteem, and can have long-term effects on a person's mental health and social functioning.

Academic pressure: Excessive pressure to achieve academically can create a sense of constant stress and anxiety, leading to feelings of inadequacy and fear of failure.

Social rejection or exclusion: Experiencing rejection or exclusion from peers can be deeply hurtful and can contribute to feelings of loneliness, low self-worth, and depression.

As you explore the roots of your own childhood trauma, remember that everyone's experiences are unique. It's possible that your trauma may stem from a combination of factors or experiences that don't fit neatly into any single category. The key is to approach your exploration with curiosity, compassion, and openness, allowing yourself to uncover the hidden aspects of your past that may be affecting your present.

In the next chapter, we will delve into how unresolved childhood trauma can impact various aspects of your relationships, from intimate partners to friends and colleagues. By understanding these connections, you can begin to unravel the complex web of emotions and patterns that have shaped your life, and ultimately, take steps toward healing and transformation.

Chapter 8

Unresolved childhood trauma can significantly impact our relationships with others, influencing the way we connect, communicate, and show love.

In this chapter, we'll explore the ways in which trauma can affect different types of relationships, including intimate partnerships, friendships, and work or professional relationships.

Intimate Partners

Childhood trauma can shape our beliefs and expectations about love, trust, and safety in romantic relationships. Some common ways that trauma may influence our intimate partnerships include:

Fear of intimacy: Those who have experienced trauma may fear vulnerability, as it can evoke feelings of helplessness or the fear of being hurt again. This may lead to emotional distancing, making it difficult to form deep, meaningful connections.

Attachment issues: Trauma can disrupt our ability to form secure attachments, leading to patterns of anxious, avoidant, or disorganized attachment in adult relationships. This can manifest as clinginess, fear of abandonment, or difficulty trusting others.

Communication challenges: Unresolved trauma can hinder open and honest communication, as it may be difficult to express emotions, needs, or boundaries, for fear of rejection or criticism.

Friendships

Our friendships can also be affected by unresolved childhood trauma. Here are some ways trauma may influence our connections with friends:

Difficulty forming and maintaining friendships: Trauma can create barriers to forming new friendships or sustaining existing ones, as trust and vulnerability may be challenging.

People-pleasing tendencies: In an attempt to gain acceptance and avoid rejection, those with unresolved trauma may adopt a people-pleasing attitude, neglecting their own needs and desires.

Attraction to toxic friendships: Unresolved trauma may lead individuals to seek out relationships that mirror their past experiences, perpetuating a cycle of unhealthy connections.

Work and Professional Life

Trauma can also have an impact on our professional relationships and work environment. Some examples include:

Imposter syndrome: Unresolved trauma can contribute to feelings of self-doubt and inadequacy in the workplace, making it difficult to recognize and celebrate one's own achievements and abilities.

Difficulty with authority figures: Traumatic experiences involving authority figures in childhood, such as parents or teachers, can create challenges when interacting with supervisors or managers in the workplace.

Conflict avoidance: Fear of confrontation or rejection may lead individuals with unresolved trauma to avoid addressing issues or conflicts in the workplace, potentially hindering their professional growth and success.

Recognizing the ways in which unresolved childhood trauma affects various aspects of our relationships can provide valuable insights into the patterns and dynamics that shape our connections with others. By understanding these influences, we can begin to address the underlying issues, cultivate healthier relationship patterns, and ultimately, foster deeper, more fulfilling connections.

In the next chapter, we will explore strategies for healing from childhood trauma, including self-compassion, seeking support, and using mindfulness and grounding techniques. By taking steps toward healing, you can begin to unravel the trauma web and create a more empowered, connected future.

Chapter 9

Embarking on the journey of healing from childhood trauma is a courageous and transformative process. As you begin to acknowledge and confront your past experiences, it's essential to equip yourself with effective strategies to support your healing journey. In this chapter, we'll explore some key approaches that can help you overcome childhood trauma and create a brighter, more resilient future.

Cultivating Self-Compassion

One of the most important steps in healing from trauma is learning to be kind and gentle with yourself. Self-compassion involves acknowledging your own pain and suffering, and offering yourself the same care and understanding that you would give to a loved one in need.

To practice self-compassion, try to be aware of your internal dialogue and challenge any self-critical thoughts or judgments. Remind yourself that healing is a process and that it's okay to stumble or feel overwhelmed at times. Be patient with yourself, and remember that you are deserving of love and support.

Seeking Professional Support

Working with a mental health professional, such as a therapist or counselor, can be an invaluable resource in your healing journey. A trained professional can help you explore your past experiences, identify patterns and beliefs that may be holding you back, and provide guidance and support as you navigate the challenges of healing.

When seeking professional support, it's important to find a therapist who specializes in trauma and with whom you feel comfortable and safe. Remember that it's okay to shop around and meet with several therapists before choosing the one who feels like the best fit for you.

Building a Support Network

In addition to professional support, it's essential to surround yourself with friends, family members, or support groups that understand and support your healing journey. A strong support network can provide encouragement, a listening ear, and a safe space for you to express your thoughts and feelings.

To build your support network, consider joining a trauma survivors' group, engaging in online forums or support communities, or simply reaching out to friends and family members who are understanding and empathetic.

Mindfulness and Grounding Techniques

Mindfulness and grounding techniques can help you stay present and connected to your body, even when experiencing difficult emotions or memories. By focusing on your breath, physical sensations, or your surroundings, you can create a sense of calm and stability amid the challenges of healing.

Some mindfulness and grounding practices to consider include deep breathing exercises, progressive muscle relaxation, visualization, or engaging in activities that bring you joy and help you feel connected to the present moment.

Establishing Healthy Boundaries

Learning to set and maintain healthy boundaries is a crucial aspect of healing from childhood trauma. Establishing boundaries involves clearly communicating your needs, limits, and expectations in your relationships, and respecting the boundaries of others.

As you work on setting boundaries, remember that it's okay to prioritize your well-being and say "no" when necessary. By establishing healthy boundaries, you can create a supportive and nurturing environment that fosters your healing and growth.

Healing from childhood trauma is a journey that requires patience, courage, and self-compassion. As you explore these strategies and find what works best for you, remember that each step you take brings you closer to a life free from the invisible shackles of your past.

With time, perseverance, and support, you can overcome your childhood trauma and create a future filled with connection, resilience, and inner peace.

Chapter 10

As you progress on your healing journey, it's essential to focus on nurturing resilience—the ability to adapt and thrive in the face of adversity. By developing resilience, you can build a stronger, more empowered version of yourself, better equipped to handle life's challenges and embrace personal growth. In this chapter, we'll explore strategies for fostering resilience and cultivating a mindset that promotes healing and transformation.

Embracing Self-Awareness

Developing self-awareness is a critical aspect of building resilience. By understanding your thoughts, emotions, and behaviors, you can identify patterns that may be holding you back and work towards creating healthier habits. Practice self-reflection by journaling, engaging in meditation, or simply taking time to check in with yourself throughout the day.

Fostering Positive Relationships

Positive relationships are a cornerstone of resilience. Surround yourself with people who uplift, support, and inspire you, and make an effort to nurture these connections. Reach out to friends and loved ones regularly, attend social events, or join clubs and organizations that align with your interests and values.

Setting Realistic Goals

Setting and achieving realistic goals can boost your confidence and sense of accomplishment, contributing to a more resilient mindset. Break larger objectives into smaller, manageable steps, and celebrate your progress along the way. Remember to be patient with yourself, and adjust your goals as needed to support your healing journey.

Developing Healthy Coping Skills

When faced with stress or adversity, having a toolkit of healthy coping skills can help you navigate difficult emotions and maintain your resilience. Some examples of healthy coping skills include physical exercise, creative expression, spending time in nature, or engaging in activities that bring you joy and relaxation.

Practicing Gratitude

Cultivating a mindset of gratitude can help shift your focus from what's lacking in your life to the abundance and goodness that surrounds you. By practicing gratitude, you can build resilience and foster a more positive outlook on life. Consider keeping a gratitude journal, expressing your appreciation to others, or simply taking a few moments each day to reflect on the things you're grateful for.

Embracing Change

Change is an inevitable part of life, and learning to embrace it is key to building resilience. Rather than resisting change, try to view it as an opportunity for growth and self-discovery. Remind yourself of your past successes in navigating change, and trust in your ability to adapt and thrive in new circumstances.

Seeking Opportunities for Growth

Resilient individuals view challenges as opportunities for personal growth and learning. Adopt a growth mindset by embracing the idea that you can always learn, grow, and improve, even in the face of adversity. Seek out new experiences and challenges that push you out of your comfort zone, and approach them with curiosity and enthusiasm.

By integrating these strategies into your daily life, you can cultivate resilience and empower yourself to overcome the challenges of healing from childhood trauma. As you continue on your journey, remember that resilience is not a destination, but a lifelong practice that will support your growth, healing, and transformation. Embrace each step with courage and determination, and trust in your ability to rise above your past and create a brighter, more resilient future.

Chapter 11

Forgiveness is a powerful and transformative aspect of healing from childhood trauma. By learning to forgive yourself and others, you can release the emotional burden of the past and open the door to inner peace and personal growth. In this chapter, we'll explore the importance of forgiveness, the challenges in embracing it, and practical steps for cultivating forgiveness in your healing journey.

Understanding Forgiveness

Forgiveness is the process of releasing feelings of anger, resentment, and hurt towards oneself or others. It doesn't mean excusing or condoning harmful behavior, but rather choosing to let go of the emotional pain associated with the past. Forgiveness allows you to reclaim your power and find freedom from the hold that past experiences have had on your life.

Forgiving Yourself

Forgiving yourself is an essential aspect of healing from childhood trauma. It involves acknowledging and accepting your past choices, mistakes, and imperfections without judgment. Remember that you did the best you could with the knowledge and resources available to you at the time. By forgiving yourself, you can release self-blame, shame, and guilt, and create space for self-compassion, growth, and healing.

Forgiving Others

Forgiving those who have caused you pain can be a challenging but liberating experience. It's important to remember that forgiveness is not about the other person, but about freeing yourself from the emotional baggage associated with past experiences. By choosing to forgive, you can release the toxic emotions that have been weighing you down and make room for inner peace and healing.

The Challenges of Forgiveness

Embracing forgiveness can be difficult, particularly when the pain of the past feels overwhelming. It's essential to approach the process with patience, self-compassion, and understanding. Remember that forgiveness is not a one-time event, but a journey that unfolds over time. It's okay to feel anger, hurt, or resistance, and it's important to honor and validate these emotions as part of the healing process.

Practical Steps for Cultivating Forgiveness

To support your journey towards forgiveness, consider the following strategies:

Practice empathy: Put yourself in the shoes of the person who hurt you or imagine what factors may have contributed to their behavior. This can help you cultivate understanding and compassion, which can facilitate the process of forgiveness.

Write a forgiveness letter: Writing a letter to the person who hurt you, or to yourself, can be a powerful way to express your feelings, release your emotions, and work towards forgiveness. You don't need to send the letter, but the act of writing can be therapeutic and cathartic.

Engage in forgiveness-focused therapy: Working with a therapist who specializes in forgiveness can provide valuable guidance and support as you navigate the challenges of healing and letting go.

Use visualization techniques: Visualize yourself releasing the pain and hurt associated with past experiences, or imagine a future in which you have fully embraced forgiveness and found inner peace.

Practice self-care: Prioritize self-care and engage in activities that nurture your physical, emotional, and spiritual well-being, as this can create a supportive environment for cultivating forgiveness.

By embracing the power of forgiveness, you can unshackle yourself from the past and open your heart to a future filled with healing, growth, and inner peace. Remember that forgiveness is a journey, not a destination, and that each step you take brings you closer to a life free from the emotional burden of past experiences. With time, patience, and self-compassion, you can find the freedom and strength to truly let go and move forward.

Chapter 12

Embracing vulnerability is a crucial aspect of healing from childhood trauma and fostering personal growth. By allowing ourselves to be vulnerable, we can connect with our authentic selves and create deeper, more meaningful relationships with others. In this chapter, we'll explore the transformative power of vulnerability and provide guidance on how to cultivate vulnerability in your life.

Identifying Your Strengths and Values

To embrace your authentic self, it's essential to understand and acknowledge your unique strengths and values. By recognizing the qualities that make you who you are, you can foster a sense of self-awareness and self-compassion that supports vulnerability. Take time to reflect on your strengths and values, considering the experiences and passions that have shaped your identity. Acknowledge your achievements and the positive traits that you possess, and use these insights to guide your actions and decisions moving forward.

Overcoming the Fear of Rejection

The fear of rejection can be a significant barrier to vulnerability, as it often prevents us from opening up and sharing our true selves with others. To overcome this fear, it's essential to build a sense of self-worth that is independent of external validation. Recognize that your worth is not determined by the opinions or approval of others, and that rejection is a natural part of life that everyone experiences. By cultivating a strong sense of self-worth, you can approach vulnerability with courage and resilience, allowing yourself to be seen and heard without fear of judgment or rejection.

Nurturing Self-Expression

Self-expression is a vital component of vulnerability, as it allows us to share our thoughts, feelings, and experiences with others. To nurture self-expression, practice openly and honestly communicating your emotions, needs, and desires. Explore various forms of self-expression, such as writing, art, or movement, to discover what feels most authentic and empowering for you. By embracing self-expression, you can foster a deeper connection with your authentic self and create space for vulnerability in your life.

Building Trust and Emotional Safety

To cultivate vulnerability, it's essential to create an environment of trust and emotional safety, both within yourself and in your relationships with others. Develop a strong sense of self-trust, believing in your ability to navigate challenges and make decisions that align with your values and needs. In your relationships, prioritize open communication, honesty, and mutual respect, creating a safe space for vulnerability to flourish.

Practicing Vulnerability in Everyday Life

Incorporating vulnerability into your daily life can help you build resilience and foster a deeper connection with your authentic self. Practice vulnerability by sharing your feelings and experiences with trusted friends and family members, seeking support when needed, and embracing opportunities for growth and self-discovery. Remember that vulnerability is a lifelong practice, and that each step you take towards embracing your authentic self brings you closer to healing and personal growth.

By embracing vulnerability and allowing yourself to be seen and heard, you can unlock the transformative power of your authentic self. As you nurture vulnerability in your life, you'll find that your relationships deepen, your sense of self-worth strengthens, and your capacity for growth and healing expands. Embrace the gift of vulnerability, and let your authentic self shine brightly as you continue your journey towards healing and personal growth.

Chapter 13

As you progress on your healing journey and begin to overcome the effects of childhood trauma, you'll start to experience a newfound sense of freedom and empowerment. In this chapter, we'll explore how you can embrace your new life, create lasting change, and thrive as you move forward from your past experiences.

Celebrating Your Progress

Acknowledge and celebrate the progress you've made on your healing journey. Recognize the hard work, courage, and determination that have led you to this point, and allow yourself to feel a sense of accomplishment and pride. Celebrating your progress can help reinforce your commitment to continued growth and healing.

Creating New Patterns

As you move forward, it's essential to create new patterns of thought and behavior that support your growth and well-being. Identify any lingering negative beliefs or habits, and work to replace them with healthier, more empowering alternatives. This may involve setting new goals, establishing healthy routines, or seeking out new experiences that align with your values and aspirations.

Cultivating Self-Love

Healing from childhood trauma involves learning to love and accept yourself, flaws and all. Practice self-love by nurturing your physical, emotional, and spiritual well-being, and by making time for self-care and activities that bring you joy and fulfillment. Remember that you are deserving of love, respect, and happiness, and make a conscious effort to treat yourself with kindness and compassion.

Fostering Resilience

As you embrace your new life, continue to cultivate resilience, which will support you in navigating any challenges that may arise. Practice the strategies outlined in Chapter 6, such as embracing self-awareness, setting realistic goals, and developing healthy coping skills. By fostering resilience, you can build a strong foundation for lasting change and personal growth.

Engaging in Lifelong Learning

Healing from childhood trauma is a lifelong journey, and it's essential to remain open to learning and growing throughout your life. Seek out new opportunities for personal development, whether through books, workshops, therapy, or support groups. Embrace a growth mindset, and view each experience as an opportunity to learn, evolve, and deepen your understanding of yourself and the world around you.

Sharing Your Story

Sharing your story of healing and transformation can be a powerful way to inspire and support others who may be struggling with their own past experiences. Consider writing, speaking, or engaging in advocacy work to raise awareness about childhood trauma and the potential for healing. By sharing your journey, you can contribute to a broader conversation about trauma, healing, and resilience, and help others find hope and strength in their own struggles.

As you embrace your new life and continue to heal from childhood trauma, remember that you have the power to create lasting change and build a future filled with meaning, joy, and inner peace. By celebrating your progress, creating new patterns, and remaining committed to growth and self-discovery, you can thrive and flourish in the face of adversity. With courage, resilience, and determination, you can transform your life and inspire others to do the same.

Chapter 14

As you embark on your own healing journey, you may find yourself in a position to support friends or family members who are also grappling with the effects of childhood trauma. In this chapter, we'll discuss how you can help your loved ones navigate their healing process, providing compassion, understanding, and encouragement along the way.

Offering Empathy and Validation

One of the most powerful ways you can support a loved one who is healing from childhood trauma is by offering empathy and validation. Listen attentively to their feelings and experiences, and validate their emotions by acknowledging their pain and the courage it takes to confront their past. Avoid offering unsolicited advice or minimizing their experiences, and instead, focus on providing a safe, non-judgmental space for them to share their story.

Educating Yourself

To better support your loved one, take the time to educate yourself about childhood trauma and its effects. Understanding the complexities of trauma can help you approach your loved one with greater compassion and insight. Familiarize yourself with the signs and symptoms of trauma, as well as effective strategies for healing and recovery.

Encouraging Professional Support

While your love and support are invaluable to your loved one's healing journey, it's important to recognize the limitations of your role. Encourage your friend or family member to seek professional help, such as therapy or counseling, to address their trauma more effectively. Offer to assist them in finding a qualified therapist or support group if they're unsure where to begin.

Respecting Boundaries

Healing from childhood trauma often involves setting and maintaining healthy boundaries. Be respectful of your loved one's boundaries, and avoid pushing them to share or confront their experiences before they're ready. Offer support and encouragement, but allow them to dictate the pace and direction of their healing journey.

Practicing Self-Care

Supporting a loved one through their healing process can be emotionally challenging and draining. Make sure to prioritize your own self-care and well-being, setting boundaries when necessary to protect your mental and emotional health. Engage in activities that bring you joy, relaxation, and a sense of balance, and seek support from others if you feel overwhelmed.

Celebrating Progress

Acknowledge and celebrate the progress your loved one makes in their healing journey. Offer words of encouragement and praise for the courage and determination they demonstrate in confronting their past and working towards recovery. By celebrating their progress, you can help bolster their confidence and reinforce the importance of their healing journey.

By offering empathy, understanding, and support, you can play a vital role in your loved one's journey towards healing from childhood trauma. Remember that healing is a process that unfolds over time, and your patience, compassion, and encouragement can make a meaningful difference in your loved one's path to recovery. As you support them in their journey, you'll not only strengthen your relationship but also contribute to the collective healing of those affected by childhood trauma.

Chapter 15

A strong support network is essential for healing from childhood trauma. By connecting with others who share similar experiences, you can find encouragement, understanding, and camaraderie in your journey towards recovery. In this chapter, we'll discuss the benefits of building a supportive community and provide guidance on how to find and nurture connections with others who are also healing from childhood trauma.

The Importance of Connection

Connection plays a crucial role in the healing process, as it helps combat feelings of isolation and loneliness that often accompany childhood trauma. By connecting with others who have experienced similar challenges, you can find validation, empathy, and a shared sense of understanding. These connections can provide a source of strength and inspiration, fostering resilience and personal growth.

Finding Support Groups

Support groups offer a safe space for individuals to share their experiences, learn from one another, and find encouragement and understanding. Many organizations offer support groups specifically for those healing from childhood trauma. To find a group in your area, consider contacting local mental health organizations, community centers, or conducting an online search.

Engaging in Therapy or Counseling

Therapy and counseling can provide valuable guidance and support as you navigate your healing journey. Many therapists offer group therapy sessions, which can be an excellent opportunity to connect with others who are also working through childhood trauma. Ask your therapist or counselor for recommendations, or search for group therapy options in your area.

Participating in Online Communities

Online communities and forums offer another way to connect with others who share similar experiences. Many websites and social media platforms host groups dedicated to supporting individuals healing from childhood trauma. While online connections may not replace in-person interactions, they can still provide valuable support, understanding, and camaraderie.

Attending Workshops and Retreats

Workshops, retreats, and conferences focused on healing from childhood trauma can provide an immersive experience and the opportunity to form meaningful connections with others. These events often feature expert speakers, group discussions, and therapeutic activities designed to promote healing and personal growth. Search online or inquire with local mental health organizations for upcoming events in your area.

Nurturing Your Connections

Once you've established connections with others on the healing journey, it's essential to nurture these relationships. Make an effort to stay in touch, attend group meetings regularly, and be present and supportive during conversations. By investing time and energy in these connections, you can create a strong, lasting support network that will sustain you throughout your healing journey.

Expanding Your Circle

As you continue to heal and grow, consider expanding your circle of support to include individuals from various backgrounds and experiences. Connecting with a diverse range of people can offer fresh perspectives, insights, and opportunities for learning and growth.

By building a supportive community of individuals who share your experiences and understand your journey, you can find the strength, encouragement, and understanding needed to heal from childhood trauma. As you continue to connect with others, remember that your story also has the power to inspire and support those around you, fostering a collective healing process and creating a world where everyone can find hope, resilience, and the courage to overcome their past.

Chapter 16

As you continue to heal from childhood trauma, you may feel compelled to use your experiences to help others and contribute to a greater understanding of the long-term effects of trauma. In this chapter, we'll discuss the importance of advocacy and awareness, and explore ways you can make a difference in the lives of others and promote a future where childhood trauma is acknowledged, understood, and addressed effectively.

Sharing Your Story

One of the most powerful ways to raise awareness about childhood trauma is by sharing your personal story. By speaking openly about your experiences, you can help break the silence and stigma surrounding trauma, fostering greater understanding and empathy. Consider writing a blog, creating a podcast, or speaking at events, workshops, or conferences to share your journey and inspire others.

Engaging in Advocacy Work

Advocacy work can involve raising awareness about childhood trauma, promoting policy changes, or supporting organizations that provide resources and assistance to those affected by trauma. By engaging in advocacy, you can help create a world where childhood trauma is acknowledged, addressed, and prevented. Explore local, national, or international organizations that align with your values and interests, and consider volunteering, fundraising, or participating in awareness campaigns.

Providing Support and Mentorship

As you progress in your healing journey, you may find yourself in a position to offer support and mentorship to others who are grappling with their own trauma. By providing guidance, understanding, and encouragement, you can help others find hope, strength, and resilience in their healing process. Consider becoming a peer support specialist or volunteering with organizations that offer mentorship programs.

Promoting Education and Training

Education and training are crucial components of raising awareness and understanding of childhood trauma. By promoting educational resources and opportunities, you can help ensure that professionals, caregivers, and community members are equipped with the knowledge and skills needed to support those affected by trauma. Advocate for trauma-informed training in schools, mental health organizations, and other community institutions, or consider organizing workshops and seminars to share your knowledge and expertise.

Supporting Prevention Efforts

Preventing childhood trauma is essential in fostering a future where children can grow and thrive without experiencing lasting harm. Support prevention efforts by advocating for policies and programs that address the root causes of trauma, such as poverty, substance abuse, and domestic violence. Additionally, work to promote positive parenting practices and early intervention strategies that can help protect children from the detrimental effects of trauma.

By engaging in advocacy and awareness efforts, you can play a vital role in creating a future where childhood trauma is recognized, understood, and addressed effectively. Your experiences, knowledge, and passion can inspire others and contribute to a world where every child has the opportunity to grow, heal, and thrive. Embrace your power to make a difference, and remember that your voice and your story have the potential to transform lives and shape the future for generations to come.

Chapter 17

Healing from childhood trauma is a lifelong journey, marked by growth, self-discovery, and continued transformation. As you move forward from your past experiences, it's essential to remain committed to growth and open to new possibilities for healing and personal development. In this final chapter, we'll reflect on the importance of embracing a lifelong journey of healing and growth, and offer guidance on how to continue nurturing your well-being beyond trauma.

Maintaining a Growth Mindset

Adopting a growth mindset involves viewing challenges and setbacks as opportunities for learning and personal development. By embracing a growth mindset, you can approach your healing journey with curiosity, resilience, and a sense of empowerment, allowing you to overcome obstacles and continue evolving throughout your life.

Continuing Education and Self-Exploration

As you progress in your healing journey, seek out opportunities for continued education and self-exploration. Engage with books, workshops, therapy, or support groups that offer new perspectives and insights, and remain open to the possibility of change and growth. By continually expanding your knowledge and understanding of yourself, you can foster a deeper connection with your inner self and the world around you.

Embracing Self-Care and Mindfulness

Prioritizing self-care and mindfulness is essential for maintaining your well-being and supporting continued growth and healing. Cultivate a self-care routine that nurtures your physical, emotional, and spiritual well-being, and make time for activities that bring you joy, relaxation, and a sense of balance. Additionally, practice mindfulness techniques, such as meditation or yoga, to help you stay present and connected with your inner self.

Nurturing Relationships

The connections you share with others can play a significant role in supporting your healing journey. Continue to nurture your relationships with friends, family, and your supportive community, and seek out new connections that inspire growth and understanding. Remember that you are deserving of love, respect, and support, and strive to build a network of people who uplift and empower you.

Setting New Goals and Embracing Change

As you continue to heal and grow, set new goals for yourself that align with your values, passions, and aspirations. Embrace change as a natural part of life and remain open to new possibilities and experiences that can enrich your journey. By setting new goals and embracing change, you can continue to evolve, thrive, and find meaning and fulfillment in your life.

Offering Support and Inspiration to Others

Your experiences and growth can serve as a source of inspiration and support for others who may be grappling with their own trauma or challenges. Share your story, offer guidance, and provide encouragement to those around you, and remember that your journey has the power to inspire hope, resilience, and healing in others.

Healing from childhood trauma is a lifelong journey marked by growth, transformation, and continued self-discovery. Embrace the process, remain committed to your healing, and continue to nurture your well-being, relationships, and personal growth. As you move forward, remember that you have the power to create a life of joy, meaning, and inner peace, and that your journey can serve as a beacon of hope and inspiration for others on their path to healing.